FISHY MERCURY

☿

Heavy Metal Tragedy

SAMUEL PINE

To my dear Mom,
and to all of the lovers of the sea..

FISHY MERCURY

To my dear Mom,
and to all of the lovers of the sea..

FISHY MERCURY

INSIDE

☿

PREFACE

We've been told that there are alarming levels of mercury in the ocean, on land and in the air we breath. The truth of the matter is that mercury levels are rising in certain species of fish more than others, and in those fish that eat the mercury laden fish. As long as we know what we're eating, I believe we can avoid the problem areas and still enjoy seafood as we study to find better ways of filtering pollutants.

WHAT IS MERCURY?

Mercury is an extremely rare silvery metal which takes on its commonly seen liquid form at room temperature. The element is referred to by its ancient symbol, ☿, which is also the symbol for the planet Mercury. It is referred to as Hg, atomic number 80, on on the periodic table of elements. Mercury is found naturally in very small amounts everywhere on our planet and especially mined and produced by powerful chemical synthesis today in parts of China, Russia, Spain and Italy. Like most organic compounds, at the core there is absolutely no radiation and it is part of our world, inherently not a threat to our life-giving systems. All elements have isotopes, the first 80 have both stable non-radioactive ones and potentially dangerous radioactive ones; all of the elements past atomic number 80 have only radioactive isotopes — they are all around us and there should be nothing to fear in these minuscule natural doses. Dangerous radioactivity is introduced into the unstable isotopes (variants) in any given element. Natural isotopes and radioisotopes are created from a reaction with the original element, especially from within the mineral "cinnabar" through seriously powerful situations such as a supernova which could have occurred millions of years ago, through the earth's tectonic plates squeezing together with so much energy that variants are compounded from the original base element and to medieval alchemists' tricks of the trade in combining different chemicals to cause a spontaneous reaction. The most toxic mercury isotope often found in the fat and muscle of fish and even more so in mammals that eat fish is called methylmercury. It causes central nervous system poisoning, often making the person who ingests it become critically ill and go clinically insane as many royals did while enjoying their treasured curiosities. Unless you are trying to become as "mad as a hatter" like those in the 18th century with mercury poisoning, you need to limit your intake of toxic foods, starting tonight.

WHY IS MERCURY IN OUR SEAFOOD?

Mercury is natural to our environment and has been in our air, plants and animals (at extremely low levels) from the beginning. With the industrial age came air pollution and isotopes of mercury gases billowing into the jet stream and leeching into the oceans. Even a nominal amount of mercury introduced into our atmosphere will rain into the oceans and accumulate within the food chain, from microscopic zooplankton to big bass. This build up is called bioaccumulation and biomagnification and only occurs in elements that are difficult to break down, such as mercury or DDT.

THE HISTORY OF MERCURY

Mercury has been discovered in many ritualistic archeological sites and was believed to have magical powers. Often referred to in older texts as Quicksilver ("quick" meaning "alive" in the medieval lexicon), it has been found as riches in Egyptian tombs dated at 2000 B.C. and in ancient Chinese dioramas used as brilliant flowing rivers in their art. The liquid metal has always been mysterious and intriguing to study. I remember playing with it as a child in elementary school, although I don't recall being told the important caution in that it is absorbed by the body through contact with the skin, the digestive tract and also easily inhaled as an odorless gas if heated. Silvery and shiny, as mesmerizing as the moon, Mercury has been found throughout the ages in bowls filled purely with mercury for royalty to use as mirrors, concoctions mixed by alchemists and by doctors who created blue pills to cure all types of ailments and as a disinfectant or cleaning agent. The effects on the human body have been studied so little that even as of the 1960's and beyond we've had ignorance in the handling of it. Amazingly beautiful and equally as toxic were the fountains of mercury on display at the Spanish Pavilion in the 1937 Paris World's Fair. Imagine the splendor of a water-feature using instead of water the only liquid metal known to man. Alchemists found that mercury helped as a catalyst in minerals to produce gold; in fact, this process is still used in the 21st century and many who work in the gold mining field are ill because of it. Scientists believe that we must simply stop using mercury to finally reduce the toxic levels from our food chain. As of 2015, a few nations are on board and more are subscribing to the Minamata Convention on Mercury, an international treaty on mercury usage.

SAFE MERCURY LEVELS

We are exposed to small amounts of mercury in everyday products such as thermometers, skin ointments, electrical switches and dental fillings. Dental fillings and cosmetic products with mercury are still being produced as of the year 2015 although many countries have permanently banned it. Studies have not shown any significant risk to slight casual exposure. We do see, however, small birds like the wood thrush with neurological disorders and discolored feathers from feeding off fish living in highly toxic water; their offspring have also often been born sick or with mutations. As you can see, it readily travels up the food chain from sea to land to sky. A 1950's study of birth defects by the Japanese government was conclusive in the province of Minamata where a chemical plant used mercury and had an overwhelming amount of illness. It is a fact that methylmercury poisoning causes problems in the central nervous system, heart, circulatory system and causes birth defects. The US Food and Drug Administration recommends no more than 0.1 µg (micrograms) per kilogram of bodyweight of the toxin methylmercury per day. So, for someone 66 kg (145 lbs) you would be allowed 6.6 micrograms per day as a reference rose (RfD).

WHAT CAN WE DO?

If you enjoy fatty tuna like most of us, eat your fill before looking at the charts contained herein. Seafood lovers need not stop eating fish altogether, but should be aware the potential risks and to go about their shopping consciously. Fish is good for us to eat with its high protein and omega-3 content. The biggest fish have the most bioaccumulation of methylmercury, although fortunately we can still thrive from smaller species. Tailor your intake to the most favorable seafood amounts by bodyweight using the charts below, and allow enough time in-between your indulgences of the fish that contain higher levels.

FIND YOUR MERCURY ALLOWANCE

Calculate your recommended maximum daily allowance of poison according to the FDA/EPA: 0.1 micrograms (μg/mcg) of mercury multiplied by your body weight in kilograms yields the maximum allowable dose of mercury per day. Example: a 110 lb (50 kg) human can have about 5 micrograms of methylmercury per day. Pregnant women and small children are advised to be especially careful.

MERCURY ALLOWANCES BY BODYWEIGHT
(0.1 μg/mcg multiplied by bodyweight in kg.)

POUNDS	KILOGRAMS	ALLOWANCE *PER DAY*
60	27	2.7 μg/mcg
80	36	3.6 μg/mcg
100	45	4.5 μg/mcg
120	54	5.4 μg/mcg
140	64	6.4 μg/mcg
160	73	7.3 μg/mcg
180	82	8.2 μg/mcg
200	91	9.1 μg/mcg
220	100	10 μg/mcg
240	109	11 μg/mcg

SEAFOOD REFERENCE (PT. 1)

TYPE OF FISH	MERCURY* *per 4oz.*
Clams	< 1 μg/mcg
Shrimp	< 1 μg/mcg
Mussels (Blue)	2 μg/mcg
Oysters (Pacific)	2 μg/mcg
Sardines (Atlantic, Pacific)	2 μg/mcg
Salmon (Can, Chinook, Fresh, Pink, Wild)	2 μg/mcg
Tilapia	2 μg/mcg
Haddock, Hake	2-5 μg/mcg
Crayfish, Crawfish	5 μg/mcg
Anchovies, Herring, Shad	5-10 μg/mcg
Pollock (Atlantic, Walleye)	6 μg/mcg
Catfish	7 μg/mcg
Flounder, Plaice, Sole (Flatfish)	7 μg/mcg
Scallops (Bay, Sea)	8 μg/mcg
Crab (Blue, Dungeness, King, Snow, Queen	9 μg/mcg
Squid	11 μg/mcg

* methylmercury content per 4 oz. (113g) cooked fish.

SEAFOOD REFERENCE (PT. 2)

TYPE OF FISH	MERCURY* *per 4oz.*
Trout (Freshwater)	11 μg/mcg
Mackerel (Atlantic, Pacific)	8-13 μg/mcg
Tuna (Canned chunk light only)	13 μg/mcg
Cod (Atlantic, Pacific)	14 μg/mcg
Tuna (Skipjack, Yellow)	31-49 μg/mcg
Tuna (Canned White Albacore)	40 μg/mcg
Tuna (Albacore, White, Bluefin)	54-58 μg/mcg
Lobster (American)	47 μg/mcg
Marlin	69 μg/mcg
Orange Roughy	80 μg/mcg
Mackerel (King)	110 μg/mcg
Swordfish	147 μg/mcg
Shark	151 μg/mcg
Tilefish (Gulf)	219 μg/mcg

* *methylmercury content per 4 oz. (113g) cooked fish.*

QUICK REFERENCE

These fish have the **LOWEST LEVELS** of mercury and are probably safe to eat in small amounts nearly every day:

Anchovies
Catfish
Clams
Cod (Arctic)
Crab (Domestic)
Crawfish, Crayfish
Flounder
Herring
Mackerel (Chub, North Atlantic)
Oyster
Pollock
Salmon (Canned, Chinook, Fresh, Pink, Sockeye, Wild)
Sardine
Scallop
Sole
Squid
Tilapia
Trout
Whitefish

These fish have **MODERATE LEVELS** of mercury and are
safe to eat about once a week:

Bass (Black, Striped)
Carp
Cod (Alaskan)
Crab (Blue)
Croaker (White Pacific)
Halibut (Atlantic, Pacific)
Lobster
Mahi Mahi
Mackerel (Atlantic, Pacific)
Monkfish
Perch (Freshwater)
Sablefish
Skate
Snapper
Tuna (Canned chunk light, Skipjack)
Sea Trout

The following fish have the **HIGHEST LEVELS** of mercury
and should be used very sparingly or avoided altogether.
Pregnant women and young children are definitely advised not
to eat these fish at all:

Bluefish
Grouper
Mackerel (Gulf, King, Spanish)
Marlin
Orange Roughy
Salmon (Atlantic, Farmed)
Seabass (Chilean)
Shark
Swordfish
Tilefish (Gulf)
Tuna (Ahi, Canned Albacore, Bigeye, Blue, Yellowfin)

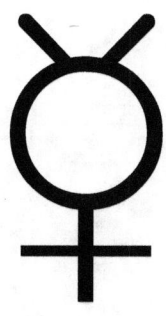

www.ingramcontent.com/pod-product-compliance
Lightning Source LLC
Chambersburg PA
CBHW071350310526
45790CB00018B/1409